Ketogenic Diet

Easy and Fast 20 Day Weight Loss Guide

Table of Contents

Introduction

I want to thank you and congratulate you for downloading the book, "**Ketogenic Diet: Easy and Fast 20 Day Weight Loss Guide**". This book contains proven steps and strategies on how to lose weight using ketogenic diet. This book is a complete resource for people who are interested in low-carbohydrate diets. It looks objectively at the mechanisms behind Ketogenic diet, which includes health benefits of the diet and offers specific suggestions on how to lose weight effectively. Diet plan meals are included and discussed in detail, which contains background physiology, together with the specific guideline, the effects of the diet on fat loss, and so much more. A huge deal of information, dealing with nutrition topic is included so that people who don't have technical background will understand the topics discussed.

Thanks again for downloading this book, I hope you enjoy it!

Chapter 1

Understanding Ketogenic Diet

Ketogenic dieting is no longer a new concept since it already has existed in many variations and in many forms. It is the same as the Atkin's diet and it is also a cousin to other famous diets such as Paleo and South Beach Diet. Are you one of those meat lovers who want to lose weight? Perhaps you might find yourself in a situation as most diets limit the consumption of meat and other fatty foods due to its high-fat calories and content. People who need to lose some weight don't need to eat lettuce and carrot sticks as they can now take advantage of their favourite egg and bacon while losing weight with the help of Ketogenic diet. Many people find it much easier restricting calories by following a Ketogenic diet. If you do this diet properly, you will consume the calories every day from protein and fats. These have been both regarded as extremely filling and quite delicious.

When you eagerly remove things such as simple carbohydrates and refined sugars from the diet, you will be able to find two-thousand calories that leave a lot of room to meet your needs each day. There are keto dieters who find it difficult consuming enough food every day.

What Exactly Is a Ketogenic Diet?

The ketogenic diet, often called as keto is a low-carb, high-fat diet, which shares lots of similarities with low-carb and Atkins diets. A ketogenic diet is a diet that requires the body of going through a process known as ketosis. The fats are usually burnt than the carbohydrates for energy. This diet is also followed properly through the consumption of high amounts of fats, low amounts of carbohydrates and adequate amounts of protein.

The human body is used to turn carbohydrates into glucose that it now sends the body the energy that it needs. When you enter ketosis by limiting the carbohydrate intake, the liver now starts to break down all fat cells into ketones and fatty acids. These are now turned as energy.

Why Does this Diet Work?

This diet works like other diets as it limits the number of calories that you must consume. This will now result to a caloric deficit whereas the body burns energies. This is mainly the fundamental science of weight loss.

With ketogenic diet that heavily relies on the reduction of calories, why do you think is there a need to cut out all carbohydrates? Why is it not ideal to just practice counting calories and concentrating further on eating a conventional low-fat-diet just like what is discussed on most diet books. What do you think is the advantage to a ketogenic diet?

So far, these are among the great questions that you would want to seek an answer for. Take note that this diet is founded with the ability to control hunger than any other diet forms. When it comes to losing weight, we always stick to a diet program that will help us make it work. We always see to it that all the diet that we follow will always bring us on the right track. We do not want to waste our time on a diet that does not bring the benefit that we are looking for. Several diet programs are popular these days and it includes Atkins, Banting, Paleo, and Ketogenic Diet. The latter is a low carb high fat diet where a person takes a higher intake of fat instead of carbohydrates. The

Ketogenic diet helps in losing weight and brings several benefits that will make an individual stronger.

Ketogenic diet provides several health benefits. Because of the low intake of carbs that produces glucose in the body, it decreases the level of the insulin and blood sugar. It helps in curing diabetes because the diet enables the body to lose unwanted fats that can be a cause of type-2 diabetes and because of this diet, several people could stop from taking medications for diabetes.

Ketogenic diet works because the foods that can be eaten also helps in losing weight like avocados, nuts, meats, chesses, and eggs. These foods contain high fat and having it on your daily ketogenic diet meal will increasingly help you reduce the weight that you have always wanted to be gone. We know that water is very important in the body but when carbohydrates are present, three times the weight it gives to the body so avoiding fruits and vegetables that are great source of water an also help in losing weight. In ketogenic diet, fruits should not be eaten because they contain sugar, which can be a contributor to weight gain. Moreover, the diet also works because it stops the body from getting hungry every hour because the high fats take some time in digesting which gives the body a full feeling and will stop it from looking for foods. Unlike from eating carbs, you usually find food after some minutes, which results to gaining weight and that is what you have been avoiding to happen.

How does the Ketogenic Diet Work?

Several people are not that satisfied with the diet since there are some who have tried the diet and were not satisfied with its results. However, there may be people who are against the low carb high fat diet like Ketogenic, the diet is effective and has helped several people lose weight or avoid themselves from getting diabetes.

Usually, the carbohydrates are the ones that supply the body energy for us to move freely and will never have to feel weak. However, when you are under the ketogenic diet, your body is more focused on eating more fat than carbs because the fats supply the energy in the body when it burns. Under this diet, you will eat limited amounts of carbs, high fats, and tolerable proteins to help you get through the day. The foods that you should eat will be more on high fat and protein and low carbs which only be gotten from vegetables that does not grow underground.

In this diet, your body will be prohibited from eating carbohydrates and should only have high intake of fats.

What Are the Benefits of Ketogenic Diet?

Ketogenic Diet has its many interesting benefits that make you more interested in it:

- **Ketogenic Diet reduces insulin spike and controls blood sugar**.

  When you eat carbohydrate-enriched foods, your blood-glucose levels usually rise rapidly. This will now cause an insulin response right through the pancreatic gland. When it comes to insulin, it will disperse blood glucose and it will cause you feeling starving again.

  When you eat a low-carbohydrate diet, you also keep the blood sugar levels steady and low. This will now result to more hunger spikes. When you reduce insulin levels, you become successful with your diet. This is also because insulin is a specific hormone that forces the body to store fats. When you just keep the insulin levels low, you create an area in your body that promotes fat lipolysis and helps limit storage of fats.

- **Ketogenic Diet Lets You Eat Food Which is Filling and Satiating**

Many people find it much easier restricting calories by following a Ketogenic diet. If you will do this diet properly, you will consume the calories every day from protein and fats. These have been both regarded as extremely filling and quite delicious.

When you eagerly remove things such as simple carbohydrates and refined sugars from the diet, you will be able to find two-thousand calories that leave a lot of room to meet your needs each day. There are keto dieters who find it difficult consuming enough food every day.

How to Get Started

Meeting ketosis doesn't occur overnight, and this isn't a form of eating, which you go halfway. If you eat in this manner, you are opting to change from becoming a sugar-burner into a fat-burner. This process takes anywhere from two to seven days, which depends on how the body adopt. The quickest way to achieve ketosis is to do a regular exercise, maintain the carb intake to 20-gram or less every day and boost the water and dietary fat intake. It is obvious that ketogenic diet could be a successful weight loss tool if you will compare it to those recommended low fat, low-protein, and high carb diets.

Chapter 2

*Ketogenic and Weight Loss and Mechanisms
Between the Two*

Evidences and studies have suggested that a ketogenic diet is proven to be effective in weight loss. This also helps lose fats, improves markers of diseases, and preserves muscle mass. There are lots of studies that compare ketogenic diet to low-fat diet for weight loss.

Even findings showed that ketogenic diet is superior even though the total calorie intake is matched. In one specific study, people who consistently follow a ketogenic diet have lost twice of their weight than a low-fat and low-calorie diet. HDL cholesterol and triglyceride levels have also been improved.

Another study has also compared a low-carbohydrate diet to the dietary guidelines of Diabetes. It was found out that a low-carb group lost 15. 2 pounds while the low-fat group lost 4.6 pounds. In just three months, the low-carb diet caused three times of weight loss.

Nevertheless, there are theories that contrast for the findings. Other researchers argued that a higher protein intake brings the results.

Others also believe that there is a metabolic advantage to a ketogenic diet.

Some ketogenic diet studies have also found out that people may lose fast when food intake is not restricted or not controlled. This is important when the research is applied to a real-life setting.

If ever you do not like counting calories, a ketogenic diet will be a good option for you. You may likewise eliminate foods and you may not track calories.

The essential point is that ketogenic diet is proven to be an effective and best weight loss diet that is supported by evidences and studies. It is also found to be very filling and it does not require calorie counting.

Mechanisms Behind Weight Loss and Ketogenic Diet

Here is how ketogenic diet helps promote weight loss:

- Higher Intake of Protein- Other ketogenic diets have been recognized in helping increase protein intake. This usually has its many weight loss benefits.

- Gluconeogenesis- The body converts protein and fats into carbohydrates for fuel. This is the process that burns more calories every day.

- Food Elimination- This helps limit carb intake and this limit the food options. This also noticeably reduces calorie intake and this is the key element for fat loss.

- Appetite Suppressant- A ketogenic diet helps you in feeling fuller and longer. This is also mainly supported by the positive changes in the hunger hormones like ghrelin and leptin.

- Improved Insulin Sensitivity- A ketogenic diet helps improve insulin sensitivity and helps improve metabolism and fuel utilization.

- Decreased Storage of Fats- Other researches strongly emphasize that a ketogenic reduces lipogenesis. This is known as the process that helps convert sugar into gats.

- Enhanced Fat Burning- A ketogenic diet increases the amount of fats that are burned throughout the day, exercise, and daily activity.

The essential point is that a ketogenic diet can be an effective weight loss tool than other low-fat, low-protein and high-carb diets. This also can help you burn more fats, reduce calorie intake, and increase your feelings of fullness than other weight loss fads and diets.

Chapter 3

Complete List of Foods to Eat Freely, Eat Occasionally, and Avoid Completely

It could really be challenging following a healthy diet specifically with the Ketogenic diet. This is also especially if you are just new to it or a beginner. In this chapter, a complete list of Keto foods will be listed for you to make the right choice. The approach is simple as it just lets you eat more real foods than low-carb foods.

What Foods to Eat Freely

You need to eat for real foods such as vegetables, yogurt, nuts, eggs, meat, and fruits. The main concept of Keto Diet is that it is not only focused on losing weight but also in adopting a better and healthier lifestyle.

Here is a complete list of the low-carb foods to include on this diet.

Wild Animal Foods and Grass-Fed Sources

- Wild Caught Fish and Seafood

- Grass-Fed Meat such as goat, lamb, beef, and venison
- Pastured Poultry and Pork, Gelatin, Butter, Ghee- These are enriched with omega-3 fatty acids
- Grass-fed and Offal

Healthy Fats

- Polyunsaturated Omega 3s
- Saturated Fats (Chicken Fat, Tallow, Lard, Coconut Oil, Butter, Ghee, Clarified Butter, Goose Fat
- Polyunsaturated Omega 3s from Seafood and Fatty Fish

Fruits

- Avocado

Non-starchy Vegetables

- Cruciferous Vegetables such as radishes, Kohlrabi, and Kale

- Asparagus, Celery Stalk, Summer Squash, Cucumber, and Bamboo Shoots

Condiments and Beverages

- Pork Rinds

- Water, Tea (Herbal, Black), Coffee (with coconut milk or cream and black)

- Mustard, mayonnaise, bone broth, pesto, fermented foods, pickles, sauerkraut and kombucha

- Herbs and Spices, Lime Juice, Zest, and Lemon

- Whey Protein (avoid artificial sweeteners, soy lecithin, hormones, and additives) gelatine and protein

What Foods to Eat Occasionally

The lists of foods you need to eat occasionally are as follow:

Fruits, Mushrooms, and Vegetables

- Cruciferous Vegetables like Green and White Cabbage, Cauliflower, Red Cabbage, Brussels, Broccoli, Fennel, Sprouts, Rutabaga/Swede, and Turnips

- Nightshades (Peppers, Tomatoes, and Eggplant)

- Root Vegetables (Spring Onion, Parsley Root, Onion, Leek, Mushrooms, Garlic, Pumpkin and Winter Squash

- Sea Vegetables (Okra, Kombu, Nori, Bean Sprouts, Snap Peas, French or Globe Artichokes, Wax Beans, Water Chestnuts)

- Berries (Blueberries, blackberries, cranberries, raspberries, mulberries and more)

- Rhubarb, Coconut, and Olives

Full-Fat Dairy and Grain-Fed Animal Sources

- Eggs, ghee, poultry, and beef (farmed pork need to be avoided as it is high in Omega 6S)

- Dairy Products (cottage cheese, full-fat yogurt, cheese, sour cream, and cream)

  Also, avoid those products that are labelled as "low-fat". These are usually packed in starch and sugar and these have less sating effect.

- Bacon- Be most aware of added starches and preservatives (Nitrates will only be acceptable if just eat adequate antioxidants

Seeds and Nuts

- Macadamia Nuts (High in Omega 3s and low in Carbohydrates)

- Almonds, pecans, pine nuts, hazelnuts, walnuts, pumpkin seeds, flaxseed and sesame seeds, hemp seeds and sunflower seeds

- Brazil Nuts (Be careful of high level of selenium- Never eat too many of them)

Fermented Soy Product

- When fermented soy, product must be eaten, only eat those fermented soy and GMO products like Tempeh, paleo-friendly coconut amines, soy sauce and Natta)

- Edamame and black soybeans that are unprocessed

Condiments

- Zero-carb Sweeteners (Erythritol, Swerve, Stevia and more)

- Thickeners like xanthan gum, arrowroot powder. (Bear in mind that xanthan gum is not paleo-friendly. This is because other people include it in their Paleo diet.

- Sugar-free tomato products (ketchup, pasta, and puree)

- Carob and Cocoa powder and dark chocolate (Better 90%)

- Be aware of sugar-free mints and chewing gums- Some have carbs

Some Fruits, Needs and Vegetables with Average Carbohydrates Depend on the Daily Carb Limit

- Root Vegetables (Carrot, Sweet Potato, Parsnip, Beetroot, and Celery Root)

- Cantaloupe, Honeydew Melons, Gallia, and Watermelon

- Cashew Nuts, Pistachio and Honeydew Melons

- Only Small Amounts of Dragon Fruit, Apple, Peach, Nectarine, Orange, Kiwi Berries, Grapefruit, Pears, Figs, and Plums

Alcohol

- Dry White Wine, Dry Red Wine, Unsweetened Spirits- Avoid these wines for weight loss as these are good for weight maintenance.

What Foods to Avoid Completely

The foods you need to avoid completely include foods rich in factory-fared meat, processed foods, and carbohydrates.

1. **Factory-farmed fish and pork**—These are enriched in inflammatory omega 6 fatty acids. Farmed fish for instance may contain PCB's and mercury.

2. **Processed Foods**—Processed foods contain MSG, carrageenan, wheat gluten, BPAs, and sulphites

3. **Artificial Sweeteners**— (Equal, Splenda, Sweeteners that contain Sucralose, Aciculae, Aspartame, Saccharin and more) These are known to cause other issues and cravings.

4. **Refined Oils/Fats**—These often consist of safflower, sunflower, soybean, corn oil, soybean, canola, trans fats like margarine.

5. **All Grains including Whole Meal (Oats, Wheat, Rye, Millet, Barley, Rice, Buckwheat, Sprouted Grains, White Potatoes, Quinoa)** These also include products that are made from grains like pizza, pasta, bread, crackers, cookies and more, sweets and sugar (HFCS, table sugar, cakes, ice creams, soft-drinks, and sweet puddings)

6. **Milk**—Only a Small Amount of Full-Fat and Raw Milk will have allowed. Milk is usually not suggested for a lot of reasons. With all those dairy products, milk is quite difficult to be digested. This is because it lacks the good bacteria and it contains hormones. In addition to that, it is high in carbohydrates (usually four to five grams of carbohydrates per 100 ml). For tea and coffee, replace milk with a cream in a reasonable amount. You could have a small amount of raw milk; however, you must be aware of those extra carbohydrates.

7. **Sweet and Alcoholic Drinks (Cocktails, Sweet Wine, and Beer)**

   You may try the healthier and better versions of popular drinks and cocktails.

8. **Tropical Fruit (Mango, Papaya, Banana, Pineapple and More) and High-Carb Fruit**

   Avoid eating topical fruits and drinking fruit juices that are one-hundred percent fresh juices. It is instead better to drink smoothies. You must remember that juices are the same as sugary water. Smoothies, however, have fibre.

9. **Soy Products**

   You must avoid eating soy products including wheat gluten that can be used in low-carbohydrate foods. When you commit yourself not to eat bread anymore, you must never dare adding it in your diet.

   Be more careful of BPA-lined cans and just replace them with BPA-free packaging like glass jars. BPA is linked to a lot of negative health effects like cancer and impaired thyroid function.

Other additives you must avoid include MSG, carrageenan, and sulphites.

Chapter 4

Understanding the Different Types of Ketogenic Diet

If you already have decided losing weight fast, you might consider following the ketogenic diet. This is a healthy diet which has already been around for years. This also has been used in the treatment of patients who suffer from seizure problems or epileptic problems including the kids.

Nevertheless, this is a type of diet that is now losing its popularity due to the advent of some prescription drugs used in the treatment of health problem. Good news, there are still lots of dieters who are follow this diet with the benefits it brings to the body.

Types of Ketogenic Diets

Beginners must first have a brief and detailed overview of this diet including its meal plan. This will help them create an informed and healthy decision in following this type of diet. Just like with other types of diet, there is also a need to consult your physician before following this diet. This is especially for those who are experiencing health problems.

Ketogenic diet is divided into three different types according on the percentage of daily calorie needs. Here are the three different types of ketogenic diet that you may choose to follow:

1. Standard or SKD

One of the first known types of ketogenic diet is the standard or the SKD. This is specifically designed for people who do not enjoy their sedentary lifestyle and who are not active.

In this type of diet, the meal plan puts a limit to of twenty to fifty grams of net carbohydrates. Vegetables or fruits which are starchy will also be restricted on this diet.

For this ketogenic diet to be effective, you must follow a consistent meal plan. Vegetable oil, butter as well as heavy creams may also be added to replace high carbohydrates.

2. Targeted or TKD

The targeted diet or TKD is less strict as compared to the standard diet or SKD. This allows a dieter to consume carbohydrates for if it will not bring unhealthy impact to the health.

This type of diet also helps dieters perform some workouts and exercise levels.

3. Cyclical or CKD

The cyclical or CKD diet is suggested for people who do some intensive exercises or weight training activities. This is not designed for beginners as it requires undergoing the standard meal plan for five days.

In addition to that, this emphasizes eating up or loading the body with carbohydrate for two days. It is always imperative for this type of diet to follow the strict healthy regimen for the most successful diet.

This is just an overview of the different types of ketogenic that you need to follow. Hopefully, you can now decide on the type of ketogenic diet to follow. If you want to obtain an in-depth and clear discussion of the different types of ketogenic diet, you need to consult your medical health provider or your physician.

With whatever type of ketogenic diet, you will choose, this will give your body an immediate and successful boost.

Chapter 5

Steps to Follow in Ketogenic Diet

Following a ketogenic diet is very easy and simple for if you are equipped with the right knowledge and skills about this diet. This diet is considered as one of the most effective and safest diets to offer immediate and successful change in your body. This is especially when it comes to weight loss processes.

If you would want to obtain healthy and successful results as far as ketogenic diet is concerned, spend all your time and effort to learn more about these steps:

Ketogenic Diet Step

There are several steps to follow considering ketogenic diet. If you really want to try this type of diet, here are the steps for you to follow:

- ### *Remove Carbs*

Check for the food labels and obtain thirty grams of carbs or even less every day. Removing carbs does not actually mean that you must eliminate them all. There are times that you need to take carbs to supply the required nutrients of the body.

- ### *Stock Up on Some Staples*

Stock up cheese, meat, whole eggs, avocados, nuts, oily fish, oils and even cream. These are the staples that could really be a part of your ketogenic diet. There are still a lot more of staples for you to buy in the market. If you don't know the type of staples to stock up, you may try consulting your medical and health service provider with this concern.

- ### *Eat Veggies*

Fat sources are known for high calorie content. Therefore, you need to add up on your plate nutritious and healthy vegetables. This will eventually help you feel fuller for a long time. There are lots of healthy and nutritious vegetables that are now available in the market today. These will supply the required minerals and nutrients of your body. Choose those veggies high in minerals and nutrients for the most successful results after.

- ### *Learn to Experiment*

Ketogenic diet can be very delicious and interesting. You might want to engage in some experiments on some of the foods to include on your everyday meal. You may as well cook ketogenic bread, pasta, muffins, puddings, ice cream and even brownies. Moreover, you may try searching for some foods as part of the diet. If you are not familiar with it, try to consult your physician first before you eat your experimented ketogenic diet.

- ### *Build a Healthy Plan*

It can be quite difficult to look for low carb type of meal in anywhere you go. This is the reason you need to design your own healthy plan that is the same with other types of diets. Your plan may also serve as your healthy guide towards eating the best ketogenic meals.

- ### *Look for Things You Love*

You may also spend some time and effort to experiment some other things that could be a part of your ketogenic diet.

- ### *Track Your Progress*

If you want to determine how successful ketogenic diet result is, you may track your own progress by taking some photos, measuring, and most monitoring your weight every now and then. If your progress stops unexpectedly, you may try to change your ketogenic diet routine.

- ### *Replace Mineral*

Ketogenic diet changes mineral and fluid balance. Due to this reason, you may add up some salt on your food or you may take some magnesium or electrolytes.

- ### *Try Taking Supplements*

To be able to boost the successful results of ketogenic diet, might as well consult your physician for some supplements to take. These supplements recommended by your physician can help you out obtain successful results in no time.

- ### *Be Consistent*

There are no shortcuts to ketogenic diet success. This is just the same as other types of diet. Nevertheless, one of the essential factors to ketogenic diet is on your consistency. You need to be very consistent in all the things you do and just stick on to eating nutritious and healthy foods for your body.

These are some simple yet most effective steps to follow when you want to obtain successful, healthy, and progressive ketogenic diet results.

Always remember that no diets are perfect for people. The diets will usually vary between body types, life styles, individual metabolism, genes, personal preferences, and taste buds.

With ketogenic diets, it can work effectively for people who would want to obtain immediate and successful diet results. All you must do is to follow the above-mentioned steps about ketogenic diet processes.

If you have already been equipped with the steps and yet you do not know how to do it properly, seek for an immediate assistance and support coming from those dieters who have been consistently following this diet. If not, you can also seek for the assistance of medical service providers to ensure that you would follow the right ketogenic diet plan steps.

How to Start a Ketogenic Diet

Now that you already know what Ketogenic Diet is, if you are already thinking about starting the diet, you need to keep in mind the below pointers. Through which you will be guaranteed with success.

1. Find and get a reliable carb counter guide – This is needed to help you learn

and bear in mind the counts of foods that have been eaten. Counting carbs is a significant part of engaging into Ketogenic Diet and it is crucial to comprehend how to do such the right way.

2. Restock your Kitchen – Doing so can help you remain on the right path. Indicated below are some of foods you should never forget when going out for food shopping. Fill your refrigerator with it.

3. Go on carb sweep – Inspect your kitchen refrigerator and cupboard, and then get rid of foods containing high amount of carb including whole grain that contains complex carbs.

4. Bear in mind that a Ketogenic Diet is not a special diet requiring special food – Meaning to say, you do not have to purchase any low carbohydrate package foods. Foods required to be eaten under ketogenic diet are essentially whole, real foods that are close to its natural state. They should not have undergone complex food processing. It is important to note that a small amount of fake sweetener pose less negative health

effects in comparison to the standard sugar amount in sweetened foods. Several people usually settle with natural sugar-alcohol sweeteners but researches have shown that those are anti-ketogenic and can hinder the ketosis process for some. The effect varies, so it helps to test it first to see whether it will affect your weight loss goal or your health in the first place.

5. Be Prepared – You are expected to spend more time in your kitchen, as ketogenic diet involves eating and cooking real foods. On its good side, people who do not know how to cook can treat Ketogenic Diet as an opportunity to learn about cooking, specifically in low carb as well as general cooking.

6. Think about meal planning – Planning the meals beforehand is beneficial as it reduces the time deciding what foods to buy at a grocery store and will give you a framework to adhere to when the mealtime arrives. If you plan to have broccoli and salmon for dinner tonight, you can avoid picking up high-carb foods.

7. Replace old, destructive habits with new, helpful ones – Preventing yourself from doing the things you are used to do is difficult. However, this step is of paramount importance if you are sincere enough about your goals on engaging into Ketogenic Diet. If you are used to eating bagel at a coffee place, try making your own coffee paired with eggs at home instead.

8. Drink as much water as you can – The purpose is to remain hydrated, which is crucial when you are under a Ketogenic Diet. When you lower your carb intake, your kidneys will begin dumping the excess water that has been retained due to the former high carb intake. Ensure to drink enough water to replace what was lost. You do not really have to follow the 6-8 glasses per day rule. Drinking water when you feel thirsty can do the trick. The lack of water and minerals like magnesium, potassium, and salt typically leads to muscle cramps and headaches.

9. Avoid foods with high carbohydrate content – These foods drive up your insulin and blood sugar levels. It is worthy to note that most individuals suffering from diet related health

problems might have suffered from untreated gluten intolerance.

10. Consider taking natural supplements – Taking supplements is not bad when you are under Ketogenic diet. Just make sure to take supplements formulated using natural ingredients.

11. Find ways to track your daily carb counts and food intake – As what the number one point indicates, you must keep your carb counts in check. In terms of monitoring your food intake, you can simply use online food intake trackers, use Microsoft spreadsheet, or simply write down in your food journal. Ideally, you should include on your tracker not only the food you eat but also the way you felt as well as the alterations you made. Through which you will be able to have a guide back in case you go off track

12. Learn how to avert your sugar cravings- If you feel it difficult to keep yourself away from sweets, you may consider techniques or supplements that can help you suppress those nagging thoughts of sweets and desserts and keep a normal blood sugar level. Through time, ketosis

can become a powerful way of suppressing your appetite towards temptingly delicious foods. Abstinence will come easier then.

13. Do not focus on your weight – You may be starting a ketogenic diet plan to lose weight but these do not mean you will focus on your weight all throughout the process. Avoid weighing yourself every other day or even every day. Doing so will not give you any accurate tracking of fat loss. Fluctuations may even just make you crazy once you focus only on your weight. An ideal pace of tracking your progress is weighing yourself once a week. Generally, instead of focusing on losing weight, try to focus on the diet's health benefits as well as long-term health changes.

14. Think about the social situations you may find yourself at – It refers to social situations where food temptations lurk everywhere such as company celebration, birthdays, and the like. However, it does not mean you should stop attending social gatherings. It is just that, you must plan what to do to handle the times when the temptations

to eat like you are used to arise. If a friend brings a box of chocolates you love at the office, or your friend offers you nachos and potato skins, you had better think of healthier foods such as steak and salad instead.

Starting a Ketogenic Diet can be difficult but being able to do so is already a great achievement. Remember the above pointers when starting a ketogenic diet to guarantee success and real result.

General Guidelines and Rules

Diet is always the answer whenever we would want to lose the excess weight that we have and achieve a fit stature. We always go on diets every time that we feel that we are gaining weight and avoid the foods that cause weight gain. Among all the diet programs that can be found around the world, the ketogenic diet is one of the most popular. A diet centers in lower intake of carbohydrates and have a high intake of fats. The diet helps the body to lose weight because it avoids the body from eating carbohydrates, which is one of the reasons why people are gaining weight since it contains sugar and starch.

When under the ketogenic diet, you must follow the guidelines and rules to make it effective. Missing just one rule can already cause a big change in your body, which can also lead you on gaining weight again. To make the diet effective, you must formulate it properly and correctly for it to act in your body and help you achieve a fitter you. However, there are also some rules in this diet that you should be aware of especially the people who are not allowed to undergo this diet program.

Here are the General Guidelines and Rules that you must follow when you are taking the ketogenic diet.

- When you are under the ketogenic diet, it is always the best decision to only eat the foods that are allowed by the diet to avoid the body from receiving too much carbohydrate. If you are going to eat other foods besides the allowed ones, always check its carbohydrates content and the serving size. Always remember that when it comes to dairy or meat products, the carbohydrates content should be 2 grams or below and for the vegetables, it should be less than 5 grams.

- When you are under the ketogenic diet and you feel hungry, only eat the foods like meats, seafood, and poultry since they are a good source of high fat. However, avoid the breaded and fried seafood and crabmeat imitations because it contains sugar and additives that can ruin the diet. Once your body is satisfied with the foods that you have eaten, stop eating!
- When in a ketogenic diet, it is always good to eat two cups of green salads every day and a cup of vegetables, which are fibrous. The green vegetables that you can include in your green salad are all kinds of cabbage, chives, lettuce, parsley, kale, chard, turnips, beet, collards, mustards, and chives. As for the fibrous vegetables, here are some that you can eat like okra, radishes, bell pepper, bamboo shoots, sprouts, broccoli, and cauliflower. It is always good to eat these vegetables when they are raw since it contains high amount of sugar and should be limited to half cup.
- When you are in a ketogenic diet, always use the recommended fats. Here is the list of fat that you should have in this diet.

- Fats that must be used when Heating or Cooking food
- Butter
- Organic chicken fat
- Organic duck fat
- Ghee is a butter where the milk solids are eliminated
- Organic lard and do not use the hydrogenated one
- Organic olive oil which is cold pressed
    - Organic coconut oil
- Organic red palm oil and should be in little amount.
- Beef tallow which came from some cattle that was fed by grass
- The fats that you should be using in cold dressings
- Macadamia oil
- Mayonnaise that encloses soybean oil
- Nuts and seed oils such as almond oils, flaxseed oil and sesame oil, which is high in omega 6
- Prevent from using vegetable oils like canola, corn, safflower, grapeseed, rice bran and sunflower because these oils have high seditious omega 6 fats that contain toxins.
- When you are in a ketogenic diet, you should eat some foods in limited amounts.

- When eating cheese, you should eat 4 ounces of it in a day since the count of carb should only be 1 gram or less in a serving.
- When eating dairy creams, you should only eat 4 tablespoons of it in a day and make sure that the dairy creams you eat do not have any added heavy cream, whipped cream, and sour cream.
- When eating vegetables that are fatty, you should eat olives 7 times a day and s for the avocado, a half of it is enough.
- When eating mayonnaise, the advisable serving is 4 tablespoons in a day and always sees the labels of the brands to check its carbohydrates amount.
- When eating lemon, or drinking lime juice, you should only have 4 tablespoons in a day.
- The ketchup intake should only be limited to 1 tablespoon a day.
- The soy sauce intake should only be four tablespoons a day.
- As for the salad dressing, it is always best to create your own dressing using oils and vinegars but not the balsamic one.
- When eating pickles, you should only have 2 servings of its dill type.

For the foods that are eaten during snacks or foods that can be baked, the pork rinds should only be in a little amount and must not be over 2 grams. The nuts and flours should only be 1 ounce a day. Do not eat snacks that contain whey protein because it surges hunger and the insulin level.

In ketogenic diet, it is not only about the food but also the beverages should also be given attention. The only allowed drinks in this diet are the clear broth, coffee which is decaf, unsweetened herbal tea, decaf team, flavored seltzer water, almond milk which should be taken 2 cups a day and water.

Ketogenic diet is a helpful diet in losing weight. In all diets, there are guidelines that should be considered and following them can help the diet become effective and will also help you achieve your goal.

Chapter 6

*Plan Your Meal Today with the Best Ketogenic
Diet Menu and Snack Plan*

Keeping taste buds entertained with ketogenic
diet is not a difficult struggle. Some high fat
and low carb dieters always find it successful
when they eat up consistent meals at a regular
basis.

Some people also tend to consider repetition of
menu plans to be difficult and quite boring to
stick with. Whether you choose to stick on
staple meals you eat every week or you want to
add up some spice on your meals, there are lots
of amazing food choices with your ketogenic
diet.

One Week Menu Sample for Ketogenic Diet

Having a ketogenic diet meal plan menu
promises you an essential and healthy lifestyle.
Your sample meal plan for ketogenic diet
should be followed on a weekly basis.

If you will start on a low carb diet, or you want
to start for some new menu ideas on your
ketogenic diet, here is a sample of basic
ketogenic menu plan best for one week.

Monday

- *Breakfast*

You can have 2 fried eggs and 2 rashers of bacon which are streaky.

- *Lunch*

You can eat green salad with grated cheese and cubed ham.

- *Dinner*

You may eat pork chop that comes along with oriental spices. You may also stir fried some spring greens.

Tuesday

- *Breakfast*

For breakfast, you may have two scrambled eggs along with chives.

- *Lunch*

For your lunch, you can have green salad with 2 hotdog or sausages.

- *Dinner*

For your dinner, you may prepare some raw or steamed spinach with sirloin steak.

Wednesday

- *Breakfast*

For your breakfast, you can have cheese and ham omelette.

- *Lunch*

For your lunch, you can have bacon and cheese with two patties of hamburger.

- *Dinner*

You can have cauliflower cheese and roasted pork belly.

Thursday

- *Breakfast*

For breakfast, you can have smoked salmon and roll ups of cream cheese.

- *Lunch*

For lunch, you can have egg mayonnaise with green salad.

- *Dinner*

For your dinner, you can have roasted chicken with broccoli.

Friday

- *Breakfast*

You may have low carb type of pancakes with syrup of sugar free maples.

- *Lunch*

You can have salami slices and mozzarella.

- *Dinner*

You can have green vegetable stirred fry with delicious chili pepper and spare ribs.

Saturday

- *Breakfast*

For your breakfast, you can have poached eggs with two sausages.

- *Lunch*

For lunch, you can have fried ground beef served with spices and iceberg lettuce.

- *Dinner*

For dinner, you can have legs of turkey with healthy Brussels sprouts.

Sunday

- *Breakfast*

For breakfast, you can have poached eggs with melted cheese and spinach.

- *Lunch*

For lunch, you can also have chicken wings which are deep fried into a lettuce bed.

- *Dinner*

For your dinner, you can have green vegetables steamed and tuna steak.

Now, you already have an insight of a simple guide on your ketogenic diet menu plan. There are still a lot more of foods you would want to eat as part of your ketogenic diet. If you are not aware of some of the healthy and nutritious foods to eat, it is always best to seek for the assistance of your physician before you plan for your ketogenic diet menu plan. They will simply guide you on the best foods to eat as part of your diet menu plan for ketogenic.

Diet Snack

Apart from the ketogenic meal plan you must have, you must also need to think of some healthy and nutritious diet snacks to help boost your successful results.

To help you out, here is the list of some of the diet snacks to have for your ketogenic diet:

- Small quantity of nuts

- Pork rinds

- Cubed cheese

- Quest bars

- Celery combined with cream cheese

- Roll up of cheese and low carbs tortilla

- Beef jerky

- Slices of pepperoni

- Cocktail sausages

- Chicken wings

- Rolls ups of cream cheese and smoked salmon

- Hard-boiled egg

As a healthy idea, you need to check on everything when considering carbohydrate content of the foods including processed foods like cheese, sauces, and sausages. There are always hidden carbs in those products used when padding out and preserving those foods. This is the main reason you need to purchase only the lowest carb choices of foods all the time. You also must count every carbs found in the food you will eat for you not to go over your limit.

You may also not eat low-fat foods. Since you will not eat too much carbs, you must only eat enough amount of fat for your energy. This is also one way for you to prevent your metabolism from slowing down as it may start on starving due to low intake of calorie.

Thus, this means to say that you must not include chicken skin and you must avoid cooking meat with fat reducing grill. Feel free to use oil and butter whenever you cook. Make it sure that you buy only mayonnaise and fat cheese. For a low-fat alternative, fat should usually be replaced by carb.

You must also drink adequate amount of water. Coffee is also good to drink but avoid loading it with too much milk and sugar. There are some sweeteners that you may choose to use but be very careful with it.

With an advanced knowledge about ketogenic diet menu and snack plan is one way to obtain immediate success in your ketogenic diet plan concerns.

Chapter 7

Proven Health Benefits of Ketogenic Diet

One of the warmest approaches ever known as far as weight loss is concerned is the ketogenic diet. This is a low carb diet designed to help your body enter the state of ketosis. Your body will burn a lot of fats as healthy fuel contrasts to glucose. This healthy state can be achieved by depriving the body with glucose by way of different food sources available in the nutrition plan of dieters.

Benefits of Ketogenic Diet

Ketogenic diet approach works for a lot of people. This is the main reason there are people who continue to show their best interest when following this type of diet.

Here is the list of some of the benefits to obtain when you choose to follow ketogenic diet over other types of diets:

1. Kills Your Appetite

Hunger is one of the single worst and unhealthy side effect of diet. This is also the main reason some feel very miserable and just give up following their diets. One of the impressive things about ketogenic diet is that it leads to reduced appetite.

With this type of diet and as you cut on carbs, your appetite will slow down. This may eventually end up eating for foods with fewer calories. This is just a manifestation that you will not feel hunger every now and then.

2. Healthy and Immediate Weight Loss

One of the most effective and simplest ways to losing weight is on cutting carbs. People who usually follow a low-carb diet tend to lose an excess amount of weight as compared to those people who only follow a low-fat diet. The carb diet gets rid of too much amount of water inside your body. With an insulin level lowered, your kidney will also start to shed off some excess sodium on your body leading to fast weight loss for only a few weeks.

You may thing that low carb is a lifestyle and is not a type of diet. To be able to succeed with this diet, you need to just stick with it. Be consistent with all the foods you eat. You also must incorporate some healthy exercises in making the result fast and successful.

3. Effective Treatment Against Unhealthy Metabolic Syndrome

Metabolic syndrome is an unhealthy condition often associated with heart disease and diabetes risks. It is usually a collection of several symptoms like abdominal obesity, high triglycerides, elevation of blood pressure, blood sugar level elevation and low level of HDL. Good news, those symptoms could be reduced using ketogenic diet.

Ketogenic diet can help reverse symptoms of metabolic syndrome that are known to be a serious and unhealthy condition.

4. Lowers Down Blood Pressure

With an elevated type of blood pressure, it is a risk factor for different types of diseases such as stroke, heart disease, kidney failure and a lot more. Ketogenic diet helps reduce your blood pressure and reduces your chances of exposing the body and life to life-threatening illnesses. If you want to lower down your blood pressure, then ketogenic diet is best for you.

5. Reduced Insulin and Blood Sugar Level

When you eat up some carbs, these will all be broken into simple sugars on your digestive tract. From there on, they will now enter your bloodstream and then elevated your blood sugar level.

With high blood sugar that is known to be toxic, your body will now respond to insulin hormone. For those who are healthy, a quick response on insulin decreases the sugar level in your body.

One of the best ways to lower your insulin level and blood sugar is by way of reducing your consumption on carbohydrates. This is simply an effective way of treating and reversing the risks of diabetes.

6. Lower Down Triglycerides

Triglycerides are known as fat molecules. These are also well-known to bring some risk factors of heart diseases. The main driver of elevated triglycerides is the excessive consumption of carbohydrates.

When you cut out on those carbs, you will notice a dramatic reduction in your blood triglycerides. This is also essential and is healthy as compared to the low-fat type of diets.

7. Excess Ketones May Not Cause Harm to Your Body

Another essential benefit of ketogenic diet is that the excess number of ketones does not cause harm to your body. All ketones that your body created are easily and harmlessly excreted by the body in the form of urine. This is a benefit of ketogenic diet since you need to undergo urine testing. This will help determine the level of ketosis in your body.

8. Burn Huge Amount of Fat

If you will follow the ketogenic diet, you will be able to improve the ability of your body to burn too much amount of fat. Apart from that, your body now can convert fat into fuel. This is also when you only consume healthy meals rich in carbohydrate. When you are in the ketosis state, your body doesn't have any other option but to just turn the fats into fuel.

9. Protein Sparing Effects

When you already have ingested the right number of calories and protein in your dietary habit, there are some things that you might experience. When you are in the state of ketosis, your body completely goes for healthy ketones than the glucose.

Since your body has huge amount of fat, there is no need to undergo protein oxidation just to produce the right amount of glucose. This only means that protein content can be used by your body for several functions.

10.   Lowers Risks of Unhealthy Diseases

All types of diets recommended for you by a medical health providers offer a lot of benefits. When it comes to ketogenic diet, you can lower your chances of obtaining diseases and illnesses.

With the many benefits that ketogenic diet can offer, it is not surprising to know that more dieters already start to follow this diet. Until these days, there are still dieters who show their great interest in this type of diet. They are mostly aware of the benefits that this diet plan could offer to them.

If you still look for the best diet to bring out the best results on your body, choose ketogenic diet today! This type of diet will offer provide you with the most successful and most progressive results beyond what you expect.

Chapter 8

Minor Flaws to Ketogenic Diet

Just like in any kind of diet, the Ketogenic diet both has positive and negative sides and it is important for you to know these things for you to have a full understanding about what you are getting into. Below are the things that will explain to you the benefits and dangers that comes together with deciding to go on a Ketogenic diet. With that, for sure, you would be able to determine whether it is the right one for you or not.

Ketogenic diet is known for its many health benefits. Despite of such concern, expect for some minor flaws. The good thing is that its benefits still outweigh its disadvantages. Until today, some health experts still argue some of its pitfalls.

Ketogenic Diet Pitfalls

Are you aware of some of the pitfalls of ketogenic diet? If not, here is the list of some of the common pitfalls that you might experience with ketogenic diet:

1. Triggers Brain Fog and Fatigue

When you seriously consider ketogenic diet, there is a possibility that you might experience brain fog and fatigue during the first weeks of the process of metabolic shift. But still, expect that your body can obtain more energy when you get into the manufacturing process of ketones in your body.

Ketones are among the main energy sources of the body. Once these have already been manufactured in your body, there will no more fluctuations in the blood sugar.

2. Altered Profile of Blood Lipid

Another major concern of people who follow ketogenic diet is the fluctuations of fat amount in the diet. This type of diet is only focused on eating healthy fats than just bacon, eggs, and butter. Statistics also indicate that shift in the profile of blood lipid lowers the level of cholesterol in the body.

3. Triggers Micronutrient Deficiency

Due to the carbohydrate restriction in ketogenic diet, you will experience micronutrient deficiency. To avoid this thing from happening, you need to focus on taking high quality mineral and multivitamins supplements twice every day. You may as well take fibre supplements for you to have a healthy digestive system in the entire process.

4. Trigger Ketoacidosis

When your ketones level skyrockets, the trigger of ketoacidosis would often occur. Thus, this can really be very acidic in nature. This only means that the blood PH is lowered. This will not be a major concern especially when you are not a diabetic. You can still be in control of your blood and your body when you allow a lot of ketones at one time.

These are only some of the common pitfalls that you might experience when you go and follow the ketogenic diet. These are not serious enough to stop you and quit on following this diet. This can always be given with immediate solution. All you need to do is to seek for immediate support and assistance from medical and health service providers.

With the increasing popularity of the said diet, adverse reactions were also reported. This includes hair loss, hypoglycaemia, kidney stones, impaired concentration, and inflammation, just to name a few. Apart from that, there has also been scientific papers reporting that undergoing long term Ketogenic diet has led to death as well in epileptic children specifically. However, it has also been stated that secondary conditions and other complications have contributed to their death as well.

On the other hand, one would be able to spare themselves from such dangers if they follow the recommendations of experts when it comes to this specific type of diet. Hence, it is important to ensure proper hydration and sufficient magnesium intake. With that, you would only be getting all the good things from your diet choice

Fallacies and Fear

Once you say fallacies, it relates to fear, which has the possible side effect or benefits for a person. Therefore, if you are experiencing this kind of situation, it is important for you to know things about fallacies and fear.

What is a Fallacy?

When you say fallacy, it is all about the appeal to fear which is a person attempts to build a support for idea by means of propaganda and deception. With this kind of action, it increases the prejudice and fear towards the competitor. The appeal to fear is usually in politics and marketing.

Appeal to fear is usually used in social policy and marketing as the method in persuasion. Fear is the effective tool to change the attitude of a person, which is moderated by ability and motivation to process the message of fear. Aside from that, it also called as a nonmonotonic which means the level of persuasion do not increase on proportion to the quantity of fear that is being used.

All about Fallacies and Fear.

Fallacies and fear is commonly known as one of the human emotion triggered thru the apparent threat. This is the minor survival mechanisms that produce a signal in our body to respond on danger with a flight or fight responses. With that, that is one of the important part our body to prevent from possible danger and keep us safe.

However, for those people who lived with a constant fear whether from corporal danger on environment or even threats may perceive, might be the cause of being incapacitated. Aside from that, this has a great impact or side effects in a person such as:

1.It can affect the thinking of a person. Once a person feels the pathways of fears, the brain will have short-circuits that has a great amount of processing paths as well as it reacts immediately into signals from amygdala. If this state is already overactive, brains will perceive the events as negative and it will remember that on that way.

The entire details of danger in environment will store in odors, sounds, time of the day, sights, weather, and other. This kind of memory is tending to be a durable even though it is also fragmented. Far along, the sounds, sights, and the other contextual information of event becomes stimuli and can trigger the fear. With that, it will bring back all the memory in fearful event and this can cause to feel afraid without the consciously of knowing why. Due to this, kind of cues that is associated of previous danger, brain can see it as the predictor of the threat. This is usually happening with a PSTD (post-traumatic stress disorder).

2.Has the Impact in Chronic Fear?

Leaving in a constant threat can weakens the immune system and it can cause of cardiovascular damage and a gastrointestinal problem such as bowel syndrome, decreased of fertility, and ulcers. Fear can be impairing in formation in a long-term memory and at the same time, it can cause damage in certain parts of brain.

Chapter 9

Ketogenic Diet Success: Exercise Tips to Follow

Ketogenic diet is one of the safest and most effective ways of losing excess amount of weight without performing any type of exercise. This is especially true as the body is in the ketosis state; each energy unit you use comes from the fat. This only means to say that when your body is at rest, it can still store the right amount of fats for you to become slimmer. This is great news for those people who are severely overweight and who do not yet start an exercise program. This is also good for people who have just recovered from their injury or are disabled.

Exercise Tips to Consider

Ketogenic diet plan effectively and immediately works only if you engage in some forms of exercises. This will simply provide you with better results than just following this diet plan without doing anything. When you have carbs and you follow some healthy exercises, it will usually take you twenty minutes to burn fat.

If you are in the state of ketosis, you will experience zero fat burning. You could potentially lose weight fast. If you will get in touch with workout or exercise program, you will have the chance to gain some leaner muscles. This will therefore lead you to burning more excess fats not needed by the body.

This only means to say that you need to adopt healthy exercise and workout regimen with a ketogenic diet plan. This will provide you with better chances of obtaining better and faster results.

If you are a novice to this type of exercise, you may engage yourself with thirty minutes of cardio exercises like swimming or walking for three times a week. You may also add up some resistance exercises to best enhance the mass of your lean muscle.

As you get fitter and lighter, you may increase the quantity and type of exercises you will perform. You may also intensify it per the capacity and ability of your body. If you are already fit and you exercise regularly, you can now perform some difficult exercises if you can do it by yourself.

Ketogenic diet plan offers a lot of benefits to your body and life without those exercises and workouts. Nevertheless, to obtain a faster and best result, try to engage with some of the best exercises.

Chapter 10

Frequently Asked Questions About Ketogenic Diet

Do you want to follow healthy ketogenic diet yet hesitant since you don't know where to start? Well, worry no more since there are already some questions you may asked in advanced that will guide you with this type of diet. Before you get in touch with ketogenic diet, it is always best to ask some questions first to your medical and health service providers to determine if your body is suitable for such type of diet or not.

Questions Asked

Here is the complete list of some of the questions commonly asked by others about ketogenic diet.

1. Can I Eat Carbs Again?

Yes, you can eat carbs. However, it is essential to remove them little by little. After two to three months, you can just eat carbs on some special occasions and you can return to your diet right after. You can only eat up carbs at a minimum amount. This is to ensure that it will

not bring serious and unhealthy effects to your
body.

2. Can I Lose Muscle?

You will potentially lose muscles as you go and
follow several diets. If you will take a high level
of protein and ketone level, you could reduce
the chances of losing muscles if you are lifting
weights.

3. Can I Build Healthy Muscle with Ketogenic Diet?

Yes, you can build muscle with this diet.
Nevertheless, this will still not effectively work
on moderate carb diets. Building muscle is
possible with ketogenic diet.

4. Why Is It That My Urine Has Fruity Smell?

If your urine smells fruity, you must never get
alarmed. This is just because of the excretion of
by-products which created during the ketosis
state.

5. My Breath Has Smell, What Shall I Do with It?

One of the common side effects of ketogenic
diet is on the smell of your breath. To avoid this

thing from happening, you must drink only a natural and healthy flavoured water. You may also chew some sugar free gums.

6. Is Ketogenic Diet Dangerous?

Some people are really confused of following a ketogenic diet or not. This is since they believed this diet is very harmful for their health. This is not true as ketogenic diet is still the healthiest and safest way of losing weight fast.

Conclusion

Ketogenic diet is one of the safest, healthiest, and most effective ways of obtaining a fitter and slimmer body. This is essential for people who are diabetic, overweight and who aim of enhancing their metabolic health. This may be less appropriate for elite athletes and for those who want to gain weight and muscle.

Just like with other types of diet, this is known to effectively work if you will stick with your plan and you become consistent always. Apart from that, this also offers a lot of benefits beyond what you expect.

Thank you for sparing time and effort to download this book! I am hoping that this book will completely help you to lose weight fast. This is the solution to your issue of obtaining a perfectly-shaped and carved body that you have ever dreamed of.

Thank you for choosing our book on ketogenic diet. Since we truly care for your needs, we will give you a chance to present your positive review with our book. It is an utmost pleasure to us to determine how you appreciate our book.

The next step is to get the courage and motivation to follow ketogenic diet.

THANK
YOU and good luck!